What Is Monkeypox

How to protect yourself and what to look out for

By

Celia Jones

Table of content

Introduction

Monkeypox is a sickness caused by the monkeypox virus. It is a viral infection, meaning that it can spread from animals to humans and can also from person to person.

Monkeypox is a viral virus transmitted to humans from animals) with symptoms similar to those seen in the past in smallpox patients, although it is clinically less severe. In 1980, With the elimination of smallpox in 1980 and subsequent cessation of smallpox vaccination, monkeypox has emerged as the most important orthopoxvirus for public health. Monkeypox occurs mainly in the central and west Africa, often in proximity to tropical rainforests, and has been increasingly appearing in urban areas. Animal hosts include rodents and primates species.

SYMPTOMS OF MONKEYPOX

There are lots of misinformation about monkeypox. We've unpacked five things to know. Monkeypox is now listed alongsidehas COVID-19 and polio on the official list of public health emergencies. A

Global Movement. Fighting COVID. Ending the Pandemic.

Symptoms of monkeypox can include:

Fever.

Headache.

Muscle aches and backache.

Swollen lymph nodes.

Chills.

Exhaustion.

Respiratory symptoms (e.g. sore throat, nasal congestion, or cough)

The initial signs of monkeypox include fever, body aches, fatigue, and sometimes enlarged lymph nodes.

The disease can cause rashes that leads to red bumps on the skin that can appear on hands, feet, face, mouth, or even genitals.

These rashes can lead to raised bumps or painful puss-filled red papules.

Monkeypox is like the smallpox virus but much less deadly.

For some persons, the symptoms of monkeypox, though painful, will clear on their own without additional treatment.

A condition called monkeypox has been confirmed in the United States and Europe, with more suspected cases worldwide.

There are over 4,900 cases in the U.S. currently, and more are expected.

Chapter one
Is monkeypox same as smallpox?

Monkeypox is a virus that is gotten from animals in West and Central Africa. Although it was confined to animals alone as previous outbreaks have shown, it can also jump to humans.

"This virus is the same as the smallpox virus; however, it's a much milder and less deadly form of it," says an infectious disease expert at Vanderbilt University Medical Center in Tennessee.

The first confirmed case was from a person who had traveled to the United Kingdom from Nigeria. Cases were noted in London but were unrelated to the first case suggesting unlinked chains of infection and there have there been no reports of death.

The rash consists of damages that evolve in the following order:

macules, or flat discolored lesions

papules, or slightly raised lesions

vesicles, or bumps with clear fluid

pustules, or bumps with yellowish fluid

scabs after which they fall off.

The symptoms of monkeypox last 2 to 4 weeks and go away without treatment.

Can people become very I'll or die from monkeypox?

Monkeypox is a mild condition according to the C.D.C. symptoms appear within five to thirteen days of exposure, but can take up to three weeks. People who get sick can experience a fever, headache, back and muscle aches, swollen lymph nodes and general exhaustion.

Some days after getting a fever, most people also develop a painful rash that is characteristic of poxviruses. It starts with red marks on a patient's face, hands, feet, mouth or genitals that become raised and filled with pus over the course of the next five to seven days. Many recent cases have involved a single damage on the genitals that do not spread to the rest of the body. Chickenpox causes a similar rash, it is not a true poxvirus, but is caused by the unrelated varicella-zoster virus.

Once an individual's boil heals, in two to four weeks, they are no longer infectious, said a virologist at the Vaccine and Infectious Disease Organization at the University of Saskatchewan in Canada.

Children and adults with immune deficiencies may have more severe cases, but monkeypox is rarely fatal. One strain found in Central Africa killed up to 10 percent of infected individuals, but there have been no confirmed deaths reported outside Africa during the current outbreak.

The identifiable rash of monkeypox, as well as its early symptoms, could be considered beneficial."The difficult thing about Covid has been that it can be spread asymptomatically or pre-symptomatically, by people who have no idea that they're infected,"Dr. Rasmussen said. Some experts say that monkeypox becomes contagious after symptoms appear, though in some cases the symptoms may be mild. There are still possibilities to transmit monkeypox in the first few days of an infection, when symptoms are not as noticeable

Chapter Two
How does monkeypox spread?

Monkeypox spreads in a few ways. Monkeypox can spread through personal and often skin-to-skin contact.

Direct contact with rashes, scars, or body fluids from a person with monkeypox, Fabrics and surfaces that has been used by someone with monkeypox.

Contact with respiratory secretions.

This direct contact can happen during intimacy which include

Kissing anal, and vaginal sex or touching the genitals (penis, testicles, labia, and vagina) or anus of a person with monkeypox.

Hugging, massage, and kissing, Prolonged face-to-face contact, touching fabrics and objects during sex that were used by a person with monkeypox which have not been disinfected.

A pregnant woman can spread the virus to the baby through the placenta.

people can get monkeypox from infected animals, either by being scratched or bitten by the animal eating meat or using products from an infected animal.

Further Definition Of Monkeypox

What is monkeypox and why is it spreading?

The virus that causes monkeypox was first discovered in the 1950s, but there are signs it has undergone changes in the past three to four years that have enabled it to pass between humans more easily.

The thing everyone should know about monkeypox is that it actually has very little to do with monkeys.
"It was first discovered in monkeys in a laboratory in Denmark, it does infect monkeys, but they're not the primary reservoir for the disease," says an anthropologist at Pennsylvania State University in the United States.
A scientist has been studying monkeypox in Nigeria for more than 15 years and was about to begin a new research project just as the Covid-19 pandemic hit. She says that the monkeypox virus originates in rodents although, it is not yet proven.
"Some scientists thought that diseases in primates were the most threatening to humans because of the close genetic similarities, "But they are realising that infectious diseases from rodents and bats are of

importance when thinking about spill-over of new diseases into human populations."

Sicknesses that pass from animals to humans are known as zoonotic diseases. Some of these can also pass from human to human once they make contact with the species.

Monkeypox has some similarities to Covid-19. But it's been there a lot longer than the coronavirus.

Further places monkeypox came from?

Monkeypox was identified in 1958 at a laboratory in Copenhagen, Demark. It was discovered in monkeys that had been imported from Singapore couple of months earlier. The first case in humans was reported in 1970 when a nine-month-old boy admitted to a hospital in the Democratic Republic of Congo was found to have been infected with the virus. Although the baby lived in an area of tropical rainforest populated by monkeys, doctors were not able to establish if he had come into contact with an infected monkey or if it came from another source. The baby recovered from the infection, but sadly contracted measles a few days later and died.

The mature monkeypox virus – is a brick-shaped envelope of genetic material, an oily membrane and proteins.

There were likely human cases before this where the virus was not identified – it causes damages that are similar to those seen in other pox infections such as smallpox – there have been cases in a number of African countries before the first outbreak in the US in 2003 when 69 cases were reported. There are thoughts that the virus was brought to the US through infected prairie dogs that had been kept as pets and housed with Gambian pouched rats that were imported from Ghana. Other cases were of people who had recently travelled to African countries and came into UK, Israel and Singapore.

But since May 2022 there have been an outbreaks reported in the US, UK, Australia, mainland Europe, and Canada. While this has worried health authorities and scientists, the number of infections in these outbreaks are a little compared to those seen in Africa, where the disease is endemic.

Where exactly this latest set of outbreaks originated is still something of a medical detective story. Genetic analysis has shown that the variant of the virus causing the outbreaks belongs to a branch of the monkeypox. There is now the suspicion among health experts that the virus might have been circulating undetected in humans, in a number of countries outside Africa for several months, if not longer.

Some genetic analysis – although still preliminary has indicated that it could have been as early as 2017 that the West African monkeypox virus picked up the ability to spread from human to human. And since then it has accumulated a high number of mutations that have made it able to infect and pass between human hosts – including one that may help it to attack some of our immune defences.

Chapter Three
How does monkeypox spread?

Unlike the virus that causes Covid-19, which primarily spreads through tiny droplets released as we breathe, monkeypox is not as immediately transmitted. It relies on prolonged close physical contact – to pass from person to person, or animal to person.

"It can also spread through contact with someone who has an infectious rash, such as lesions, scabs and bodily fluids," says a scientists, from the American Society for Microbiology (ASM). "You can also be infected by touching items that someone who's infected may have touched."

Although test on the monkeypox virus has been detected in semen by researchers, it does not necessarily mean that this is how it is spreading.

A person infected with monkeypox can transfer it to others from the time symptoms start until the rash has fully healed and a fresh layer of skin has formed. The illness lasts 2-4 weeks

Who Is At Risk Of Catching Monkeypox?

Persons who live or have close contact (including sexual contact) with someone who has monkeypox, or who has regular contact with animals that is infected, are at

a higher risk. Health workers should follow the infection prevention and control measures to protect themselves while treating the patients.

The Centers for Disease Control and Prevention estimates that about 1.6 million men who have sex with same sex face the biggest threat right now.

CDC Director told reporters on a call that gay and bisexual men who are HIV positive or those taking drugs called PREP, to reduce their chance of contracting HIV face the highest health risk of contracting monkey pox.

Newborns, young children and people with underlying immune deficiencies may be at risk of serious symptoms, and in rare cases, death from monkeypox.

People who were vaccinated against smallpox may have little protection against monkeypox. However, some younger people have not been vaccinated against smallpox because smallpox vaccination stopped in most areas after it was eradicated in 1980. People who have been vaccinated against smallpox should never stop to take precautions to protect themselves and others.

The things that put a person at a high risk of catching the virus involves close and intimate contact with another infected individual. This includes skin-to-skin contact that occurs during sex as well as cuddling, hugging, massaging or kissing. Condoms probably add a layer of protection during sex, but they can't prevent contact with scars on an infected person's groin, thighs, buttocks or on other parts of their body.

Roommates and family members in the same apartment with a person infected are also at high risk of getting monkeypox said a medical director for infection prevention at the Mount Sinai Health System.

Household members can catch monkeypox through contaminated clothes, towels and bedding. Shared utensils that has been used by an infected person should also be considered high risk, said an expert.

how can i and the others be protected against monkeypox?

 The Following steps helps to prevent monkeypox virus:

Avoid contact with people who have a rash that looks like monkeypox.

Do not touch the rash on the body of a person with monkeypox.

Do not kiss, hug, cuddle or have sex with someone with monkeypox.

Avoid touching objects and materials that a person with monkeypox has used.

Do not share eating utensils with a person with monkeypox.

Do not handle the towels, or clothing of a person with monkeypox.

Wash your hands often with soap and water or use an alcohol-based hand sanitizer, before eating, touching your face and after using the bathroom.

Those in the Central and West Africa, should avoid contact with animals that can spread monkeypox virus, usually rodents and primates.

Avoid sick and dead animals, as well as bedding or other materials they have touched.

Health officials advised people to avoid close, skin-to-skin contact with people who have a rash that looks like monkeypox

Health officials are still finding out if children and people with existing health problems are at a higher risk of the disease.

Why is it an emergency?

Health officials from several countries urged the WHO to declare monkeypox a public health emergency as the disease is spreading quickly in the past months.

From June to July, the WHO reported that cases of monkeypox had increased from 3,020 to more than 15,000. The number of countries with the virus have also gone up from 47 to 75.

Officials were concerned that the disease has spread rapidly among people who did not travel to Africa where the disease is endemic. That means it has become established in an area.

The emergency declaration brings resources and action to deal with the outbreak. It also enables countries to work together in testing and producing vaccines and treatments for the disease.

The WHO said the risk of monkeypox is "moderate" around the world, except in Europe where the risk is "high."

When you notice the symptoms of monkeypox, contact your healthcare provider for advice, testing and medical care. Isolate yourself if possible until you recieve your medical result. Clean your hands regularly.

What should I do to protect other people if I have monkeypox

To reduce the risk of monkeypox you must;
Avoid close contact, including sexual contact, with someone who is sick and may have monkeypox
Do not touch the clothes, bedding or towels of a person who may have a monkeypox rash
Avoid coughs and sneezes from a person who may be having monkeypox
Sanitize your hand carefully when visiting or caring for friends and relatives who may have monkeypox
The US increased the supply of vaccine to combat monkeypox
Smallpox vaccines can offer protection against monkeypox'
More than 15,000 cases of monkeypox have been recorded in an outbreak that has taken public health experts by surprise. This virus, which is normally a mild sickness although dangerous for people with low immune systems, has been found in most European countries, as well as the United Kingdom and Switzerland.

Do we have a monkeypox vaccine?

No, but orthopox viruses are similar, that the immune system, once immunised against one, is likely to recognise another which means that modern smallpox vaccines are likely in most cases, to prevent monkeypox infection.'

As at now, the United States has purchased 6.5 million doses of Bavarian Nordic's Jynneos vaccine, the preferred vaccine against monkeypox, and the whole supply is expected to be available by mid-2023.

Treatment given to people with monkeypox?

There are no treatments specifically for monkeypox infections, however, it is

genetically similar to smallpox which means that the antiviral drugs and vaccines developed to protect against smallpox may be used to prevent and treat monkeypox infections.

Antivirals, like tecovirimat (TPOXX), may be recommended for people who are likely to get seriously ill, especially patients with weakened immune systems.

If you have symptoms of monkeypox, you should talk to your healthcare provider, even if you didn't have contact with someone who has monkeypox.
Tecovirimat (also known as TPOXX, ST-246)
CDC holds an increased access protocol (sometimes called "compassionate use") that allows the use of stockpiled tecovirimat to treat monkeypox during an outbreak. Tecovirimat can be used as a pill or an injection.

Is there a risk of a bigger outbreak?

Monkeypox is totally not a highly contagious virus because, it requires close and physical contact with someone who is infected.
However, the WHO is responding to this outbreak as a high priority to stop further spread; for many years Monkeypox has been considered a priority infectious agent. To Identify how the virus spreads and protect more people from becoming infected is now a priority for the UN agency.
Creating awareness of this new situation will help stop further transmission.
The disease can be spread from one person to another through close physical contact like sexual contact. However, it is currently unknown whether it

can be spread through semen or vaginal fluids. However, close contact with lesions during sexual activities can spread the virus.

Rashes sometimes appear on the genitals and in the mouth, which also contributes to transmission during sexual contact. Therefore, kissing could cause transmission when there are lesions in the mouth of the infected.

These rashes can also look like some sexually transmitted diseases, such as herpes and syphilis, which explains why several of the cases in this current outbreak have been identified among men seeking treatment at sexual health clinics.

The risk of being infected is not limited to sexually active people or men who have sex with men. Anyone who has close physical contact with someone who is infected is also at risk.

Which part of the world is currently at risk of monkeypox?

The majority of cases have occurred in adult men who have sex with men, experts say that there are signs the virus may branch out of this community.
Can Children have Monkeypox?

It possible and expected, to see infections in children, health experts say. But it won't be like the other common viruses.

We are not really expecting the childcare settings and schools to see a lot of monkeypox infections run through kids," said an assistant professor of pediatrics and a medical director of pediatric infection prevention at Duke University Medical Center, "But it is possible for children to get infected."

The World Health Organization and CDC said children are more prone to this disease and complications from monkeypox compared to teens and adults, particularly those younger than 8 years old.

Chapter four
Monkeypox symptoms in children

This virus symptoms usually start within three weeks of exposure, according to the CDC. They include fever, cold, swollen lymph nodes, exhaustion, muscle aches and backache, headache, respiratory problems, and a rashes.

In this current outbreak, the rash has often been located on or near the genitals or anus of an adult, but it can also appear on other areas, such as the hands, feet, chest, face or mouth. Some people experience flu-like symptoms and then develop a rash one to three days later. Some people develop the rash first then later fall sick while other develop just the rashes.

Risk of Monkeypox During Pregnancy?

Monkeypox virus can be transmitted from the mother to the fetus during pregnancy or to the newborn due to the close contact during and after birth. Adverse pregnancy cases ranging from pregnancy loss and stillbirth, have been reported as cases of confirmed monkeypox infection during pregnancy.

Monkeypox cases are increasing in the U.S. but there are very few cases among pregnant women, which is good, but makes it difficult to know exactly how vulnerable pregnant women are to the virus.

What is known about monkeypox is that some pregnant women have experienced pregnancy loss and preterm delivery while infected with the virus. However, because of the low case counts among pregnant women, it's unclear whether these complications are high among pregnant women with monkeypox.

You shouldn't panic, but up to date with the latest health information and to talk with your provider if you're pregnant.

Symptoms of monkeypox in pregnancy

The symptoms of monkeypox are similar in those who are pregnant and those who are not., Monkeypox causes fever and chills, headaches, full-body aches, congestion, cough, and a sore throat commonly.

The common symptom that sets monkeypox apart from other viruses is a rash found on or around genitals and the anus. The rash can show up on the hands, feet, face, or torso.

Although It isn't uncommon to experience a rash during pregnancy. In fact, many women experience eczema, dermatitis, or pruritic urticarial papules and plaques of pregnancy, during pregnancy.

If you have a rash while you're pregnant, it might and might not be as a result of monkeypox it is always good to talk to your provider about new symptoms, like a rash, when you're pregnant.

Chapter Five
How is monkeypox treated in pregnancy?

Some cases of monkeypox are mild and resolve on their own without any treatment within 2 to 3weeks. However, pregnant women are considered at high risk, so treatment is recommended.

Treatment of monkeypox includes two antiviral medications and one vaccinia immune globulin. These medication have been used in the past to treat both monkeypox and smallpox. There are limited studies of Studies of monkeypox in pregnant women but in animal studies it appears that at least one of the drugs is safe for the fetus. While this globulin has not been studied specifically in the pregnant population, other similar immunoglobulins are used for various conditions and appear to be safe.

Your provider can walk you through your treatment options, so you can make your decision based on your circumstances. They will discuss the possible risks you and your baby is having, so you can weigh them against any risks involved in treatment.

How to reduce the risk of getting monkeypox while pregnant

Avoiding your exposure to the virus is the best way to prevent the virus during pregnancy. It is necessary to avoid contact with individuals and pets who have the virus, and also steer clear of anyone with an undiagnosed rash.
Regular handwashing help to prevent the spread, and the practice of safe sex is advisable even when pregnant by doing so you can help lower the transmission of monkeypox.

The bottom line?

Right now, monkeypox virus in pregnancy is uncommon, and observing these precautionary measures can help lower your risk of getting it. But if you contract yhe virus, your provider can walk you through treatment options like, how your labor and delivery might change, and what to expect if you're planning to breastfeed.

Why was monkeypox declared a public Emergency?

The U.S. Declares Monkeypox a Public Health Emergency, this announcement came as the nationwide case counts has reach 7,000.

The Biden administration declared monkeypox a public health emergency releasing up more resources to combat the disease and expanding the CDC's ability to share datas and reports

"We are ready to take our response to the next level in addressing this virus and we advice every American to take monkeypox seriously," said Xavier Becerra, the Health and Human Services secretary, during a press briefing.

A Public Health Declaration allows the Secretary of Health and Human Services (HHS) to take certain actions to talk about the threat to public health from a disease or a crisis of any kind. Public health emergencies aren't just declared in the event of disease outbreaks such as Covid-19 and monkeypox. For example, in 2017, President Trump declared the "opioid crisis" to be a "public health emergency."

Importantly, a public health emergency declaration enables for the release of resources for an actual (or emerging) public health crisis. In the case of monkeypox, the federal government can now significantly allow and check the production and availability of vaccines, expand testing capacity, and make it more convenient. It also facilitates coordination among federal, state, and local authorities, in relation to improving access to testing and treatment. Furthermore, funding is directed at coordinating awareness and prevention outreach campaigns that targets members of the communities at a higher risk and the public at large, thereby curbing the spread of the virus.

Despite the similarities between the technology used to detect monkeypox and Covid-19, there are several differences. First, the virus that causes Covid-19 is most commonly found in the respiratory tract,that is the nose, throat and lungs, whereas monkeypox virus is most found in the skin (rash). So, if someone is suspected of having monkeypox, their physician will use a swab to collect cells from the rash and then send the swab to a testing lab.

Conclusion
Will there be a home test for monkeypox?

We will soon have access to a home tests for monkeypox Over the past years, there has been a the availability of at-home tests to diagnose Covid-19. People even have the option of ordering free antigen tests that will be shipped directly to their home.

Will a home tests for monkeypox soon become a reality?

The short answer is maybe. Most home tests are antigen-based, meaning they test for a protein that is present in the sample. This tests look for a protein, rather than viral DNA, they are less sensitive than PCR tests. Meaning that an antigen test could be negative even while the person being tested has the disease.

The lab will first separate any monkeypox virus DNA from the cells and proteins that are also present, the PCR test then "looks for" a small piece pof the DNA that is unique to virus and if present, that specific region of the virus' genome is copied thousands, and millions, of times. Every time a new copy is made, a signal of light is produced, which generate enough light for the PCR test to be positive.

Another difference is that PCR and antigen tests have been used extensively throughout the Covid-19 pandemic to know people who were infected but it lack the ability to identify the symptoms of the disease. In contrast, monkeypox is not known to be transmitted from those who lack the symptoms, so it is on probability that asymptomatic testing will be common as the monkeypox outbreak unfolds.